HABIT IS EASY! AN INTRODUCTORY GUIDE

NORMAN BINGHAM

ISBN: 9798374250442

CONTENTS

I INTRODUCTION

Have you at any point considered how frequently you've messed up the same way again and again? Your habits are the aftereffect of deep rooted programming. But, a considerable lot of those equivalent slip-ups appear in your life endlessly time once more. This examination based guide will assist you with distinguishing your habits and carry on with an enabled, intentional life as you figure out how to develop better ones.

The vast majority who begin to foster solid habits, do as such with a touch of trouble and outside help. We are talking as a matter of fact! Through this program you will figure out how to assemble these habits all alone. We know it's not excessively complicated, but rather things have gotten so distressing in our lives that we want a little assistance from time to time. This course will show you how to help began making positive change through basic and successful methods.

2 WHAT IS HABIT?

A habit is an inclination to follow through with something, whether unsafe or wellbeing advancing.

A positive routine will assist you with arriving at your objectives, create both by and by and expertly, and feel satisfied. Be that as it may, not all habits are great.

Habits Are Driven By Remuneration Looking for Systems In The Cerebrum. They're frequently set off by something explicit. For example, strolling past a bistro and smelling espresso beans can set off you to need a cup. Feeling worried working can set off you to smoke a cigarette.

Inevitably, habits become a redundant piece of your way of life.

Here are a few different instances of habits:

- Cleaning your teeth subsequent to eating a feast
- Putting on your safety belt when you get inside a vehicle
- Drinking a glass of wine when you return home from work
- Eating sweet or pungent food varieties when you're focused on working

- Squirming with your note pad during a gathering

Shaping Propensities Is The Cerebrum's Approach To Being More Effective. Taking everything into account, the more assignments you can finish without with nothing to do contemplating them, the better.

Furthermore, our cerebrum's propensity toward effectiveness can be positive.

For example, drinking a green smoothie each day helps your wellbeing. Also, not relearning how to drive your vehicle consistently implies you have dependable transportation.

Obviously, this proficiency can likewise be negative.

For example, gnawing your nails each time you have a gathering at work can unleash destruction on your nails. Or then again not cleaning your teeth in the wake of eating can prompt tooth rot.

3 HABITS AND ROUTINES

WHAT'S THE DIFFERENCE BETWEEN HABITS AND ROUTINES?

The principal distinction between a habit and a routine is mindfulness. Both are customary, rehashed activities. Be that as it may, while habits run on autopilot, schedules are deliberate.

Schedules need conscious practice, or they'll ultimately vanish. Be that as it may, a habit occurs with practically zero cognizant idea.

For example, an appreciation practice requires expectation and exertion. It won't run on autopilot. The equivalent is valid for work out. You won't begin practicing on autopilot. In any case, (on the off chance that you have the habit), you'll snatch a cigarette on autopilot.

For a daily practice to transform into a habit, the conduct should occur with practically zero idea. For example, suppose you add drinking green juice to your morning schedule. On the off chance that one day you awaken and make green juice without any hesitation, you can think of it as a propensity.

4 THE SCIENCE OF HABITS

How Do Habits Shape?

Habit framing is the cycle where ways of behaving become programmed. It tends to be a deliberate cycle, or it can happen impromptu.

For example, you were in all likelihood educated to clean up as a kid. What's more, inevitably, cleaning up became programmed. It wasn't purposeful — it occurred after bunches of redundancy.

Regardless of what your identity is or what your objectives might be, shaping positive routines is a significant piece of life. There is nobody size-fits-all approach with regards to making habits, yet here are a simple methods for beginning shaping and adhering to beneficial routines.

To begin with, begin little. Try not to attempt to take on a lot on the double. Begin with a straightforward habit that you can do consistently, such as recording three things you are thankful for or requiring a couple of moments every day to ponder.

Second, find a pal or a gathering of companions who share similar objectives. Having individuals to keep you roused and responsible will make it simpler for you to adhere to your habits.

Third, reward yourself. After you've finished your habit for the afternoon, give yourself a little prize like a piece of dim chocolate or a loosening up bubble shower. This will assist you with recalling that it's worth the effort to keep up your positive routines.

Fourth, keep tabs on your development. Record the habits you've made, and monitor how frequently you complete them. This will provide you with a feeling of achievement, and help

At Last, show restraint. Fabricating positive routines takes time, and it's critical to be delicate with yourself assuming that you goof. Try not to surrender - it simply implies you want to rehearse somewhat more.

5 THE VITAL NINE CATEGORIES OF HABIT

Habits are the undetectable engineering of daily existence, and a huge component of bliss. Around a little less than half of what we do every day is molded by habits, and in the event that we have habits that work for us, we're substantially more liable to be content, sound, useful, and imaginative.

The habits individuals most frequently need to develop fall into nine regions, the Imperative Nine:

1. Energy: exercise and rest

- Hit the hay at a specific time each night
- Take an everyday walk
- Practice no less than multiple times every week
- Peruse for 30 minutes before bed
- No caffeine after a specific time

2. Efficiency: center, work, progress

- State "morning pages" consistently

- Hold a specific day of the week as a gathering free day
- Pursue a language-learning application and do the activities recommended
- Switch off the web for two hours every evening

3. Connections: associate and extend

- Read to kids each night
- Begin a gathering to examine an alternate digital broadcast every month
- Plan a week after week call with guardians
- Plan Friday date evenings

4. Re-energizing: unwind and rest

- Peruse 20 minutes per day
- Plan breaks over the course of the day
- Play guitar for 30 minutes every day
- Go to a week by week yoga class
- Lay down for an everyday rest

5. Request: clear and coordinate

- Make your bed each day
- Endure 10 minutes cleaning up before bed
- Follow the "one-minute rule."
- Every month, give things you don't need or utilize any longer
- Partake in a "purchase nothing" month

6. Reason: reflect, recognize, lock in

- Keep an everyday diary
- Ponder each day
- Volunteer one time each month
- Begin every morning with an otherworldly perusing
- Manure or dispose of single-use plastics

7. Innovativeness: Learn, practice, play

- Take a craftsmanship class
- Investigate another area each Saturday
- Sew while sitting in front of the television
- Each Sunday, watch an exemplary film
- Go to two live exhibitions a month

8. Careful Utilization: eating, drinking, spending, looking over

- Take drug everyday, before first mug of espresso
- Limit online entertainment to 30 minutes of the day
- Plan feasts for the week
- Track spending for a month
- Trade evening espresso for green tea
- Limit cocktails to the end of the week

9. Careful Speculation: save, support, insight

- Give every month to a reason you care about
- Put resources into hardware to make practice more advantageous
- Save a specific sum every month toward movement
- Spend something like 3 hours out of every week in nature

Obviously, a similar habit could fulfill various goes for the gold. For one individual, yoga may be a type of activity; for another person, a wellspring of mental rest; for another person, an act of profound commitment. Furthermore, individuals esteem various habit. For one individual, coordinated documents may be a significant device for imagination; someone else tracks down motivation in irregular juxtapositions.

In the event that you don't know, don't stress over picking the "right" class for a point you need to seek after. There's no right classification for any habit or point.

6 CHANGING HABITS: 5 MISTAKES TO AVOID

The following are five mix-ups to stay away from when you need to supplant a current propensity with another:

1. You're not controlling your current circumstance

Neglecting to control your current circumstance is one of the greatest dangers to making progress with an old propensity.

On the off chance that you're actually going to snatch inexpensive food with colleagues following a terrible day, you most likely won't stop pressure eating and take on instinctive eating. All things being equal, select to spend time with companions at an alternate area like a bistro or a recreation area.

The equivalent is valid for any habit. Ensure your current circumstance upholds the progressions you need to make.

2. You're too centered around the result

Such a large number of us center around momentary outcomes, such as shedding 10 pounds for an ocean side excursion or setting aside barely sufficient cash for another PC. However, the way to enduring change is a way of life change. Rather than zeroing in on transient results, center around adjusting your way of life.

3. You're not dedicated to propensity change

A solid propensity takes time and reiteration to shape. This implies being patient and giving yourself a chance to accomplish your objectives. Keep in mind, it takes between 18 to 254 days to shape another propensity.

4. You're attempting to make progress with such a large number of habits

Zeroing in on such a large number of conduct changes without a moment's delay can cause you to feel overpowered and restless. As we referenced before, in the event that an activity requires more exertion than you're willing to place in, you will not make it happen.

All things considered, center around transforming each conduct in turn. When that habit becomes strong, continue on toward the following way of behaving.

5. You accept little changes don't make any sense

In some cases we abandon making progress with a propensity before we even beginning. We expect that we'll have to roll out uncommon improvements that are excessively troublesome. However, consistently, we get the opportunity to improve or somewhat more terrible.

Rather than stressing over the higher perspective, begin with little, reasonable changes. When those little changes have become natural, you can gradually make greater ones.

7 BENEFICIAL ROUTINES FOR A FRUITFUL LIFE

BENEFICIAL ROUTINES EVERYONE NEEDS FOR PROGRESS!

This rundown of positive routines will work well for you whether you are a parent, understudy, business visionary or simply a customary individual. Learning these habits currently will assist everybody with excelling throughout everyday life.

1. Get On A Decent Timetable.

We want design and routine in our lives. Our bodies anticipate it. They perform best when we work on an ordinary timetable. We particularly need to eat and rest about a similar time every day. In the event that you are the parent of a small kid, you must show this propensity early. This standard stays with an individual their entire life and assists them with growing great work propensities. Track down a timetable that works for yourself and stick to it!

2. Eat A Sound Eating Regimen.

Our minds need the right food to perform at their pinnacle. Try not to go to the everyday schedule while starving. Understudies need to prepare themselves right on time to eat a fair and sound eating regimen. We will generally convey the propensities we realize when we are youthful forward with us for the vast majority of our lives. Figuring out how to eat right presently can stay away from numerous medical problems not too far off.

3. Watch Out For Your Profound Necessities.

We can't overlook our otherworldly requirements and really carry on with a full and remunerating life. We should perceive that there is a higher power and seek after our confidence consistently. We may not practice our convictions in the very same manner, yet I urge you to find what works for yourself and investigate it to it's profundities. A strong otherworldly life will work well for you.

4. Regard Authority.

Inability to regard those in power positions can prompt a wide range of issues throughout everyday life. It doesn't make any difference whether it is your chief, a cop, or a college senior member. Individuals in power have something important to take care of and frequently endeavored to get into the position they are in. They should be treated with legitimate habits and love. Figuring out how to say, "OK ma'am" and "Yes sir" will get you seen in a positive way.

5. Figure Out How To Work Out.

We want active work to remain sound. The advantages of ordinary activity are legitimate. We really want to find work-out schedules that are tomfoolery and match our singular preferences. Fostering a decent work-out routine is a propensity that will increment both the amount and nature of your life.

6. Practice Appreciation.

It is so natural to get in the negative behavior pattern of begrudging what others have. The grass frequently appears to be greener on the opposite side of the wall. Learning gratitude is indispensably significant. Work on pondering the things you must be grateful about. I do this with my little girl each night when I put her to sleep. I request that she review the beneficial things that happened that day. We then require a couple of moments and express gratefulness for those things. This helps us both to prepare ourselves to be thankful.

7. Be Reliable.

Showing up on time means quite a bit to one's prosperity. Individuals generally notice when you are late. It is a mark of whether you are genuinely serious about what you say and can be relied upon. Try not to bring uncertainty about this into individuals' brains by making an appearance later than anticipated. Make the propensity for being dependable now and you will not need to stress.

8. Be A Normal Peruser.

Being a decent peruser is an expertise that frequently isolates the great understudies from those that battle. Turning into a decent peruser takes practice. The more you read and are perused to, the better you get. Perusing has various advantages. It assembles one's jargon, extends the creative mind, and revives innovativeness. Make perusing an everyday practice!

9. Foster Great Review Propensities.

Concentrating successfully is an expertise. Individuals that carry on with life to the fullest are deep rooted students. They try constantly new things. One necessities to study and accumulate new information in a successful and effective way. Figuring out how to study and secure the information to succeed doesn't simply happen normally. It should be educated. Take a review abilities course or ask others for tips on further developing your review propensities.

10. Never Surrender!

I was let in school know that, "Champs never quit and weaklings always lose." I think this is a Vince Lombardi statement and it is unquestionably obvious. It takes determination in life to partake in any sort of accomplishment. I additionally recollect hearing, "Whenever difficulties arise, the extreme get moving." These maxims return to personal consistently when I want to surrender. Steadiness is a propensity. One can be grown very much like some other.

11. Request What You Need.

Foster the propensity for requesting what you need. By what other method would you say you will get it? It is actually basic. Frequently, when I ask, I'm astonished at how rapidly I get precisely very thing I needed. Simply check this one out. In the event that you are a parent, help your kids to ask others for what they need. This is really a conduct you need to normally come. It will assemble certainty and confidence that will serve your children until the end of time!

12. Continuously Come Clean!

Reality frequently comes out regardless of whether we need it to. Lying commonly entangles what is going on and makes us look awful. Take a gander at the outrages a large number of our legislators fall into in light of the fact that they neglect to concede reality. It is greatly improved to simply foster the propensity for coming clean in any event, when it is troublesome. This will save you a great deal of grief and hopelessness throughout everyday life.

13. Oversee Cash Carefully.

For what reason don't they show a decent individual accounting class in school? Understudies need to figure out how to acquire, save, financial plan, track, and carefully burn through cash to find lasting success throughout everyday life. Great cash propensities can never begin too soon. There are a great deal of good assets out there to help. I suggest investigating what Dave Ramsey brings to the table for different ages. Obviously, you can likewise find a ton of fabulous cash tips understanding web journals!

14. Regard The Climate.

It is by all accounts hip to be "green", however being a decent steward of our current circumstance is truly not unreasonably new. Insightful guardians have been showing these standards to their youngsters for a very long time. We just have this one world and we rely upon it for our endurance. Each individual requirements to do their part to safeguard what we have. Foster propensities now that will assist you with being a decent ecological resident for a lifetime!

15. Practice Great Cleanliness.

You truly can dress for progress! Propensities like cleaning your teeth two times per day and cleaning up consistently add to wellbeing, yet in addition lead to schedules that give one a more honed appearance. Initial feelings are strong and are generally gotten from the manner in which an individual looks. Like it or not this is valid. Begin today to guarantee you take the necessary steps to have an enduring decent effect.

16. Experience The Brilliant Rule.

"Do unto others... " is a rule we ought to all observe. Consider the contention and misfortune that might have been stayed away from in the event that individuals essentially applied the Brilliant Rule in the entirety of their connections. In the event that we practice this all the time, we will make much more progress throughout everyday life. Regarding individuals of all races and convictions is a sign of making every moment count.

17. Make Progress Toward Greatness!

For what reason finish a work on the off chance that you won't get everything done as well as possible? We want to foster the propensity for doing our absolute best. Greatness ought to be the standard we take a stab at in all we do. We can't begin letting ourselves or our youngsters do the most un-conceivable to squeeze by. In the event that we do, they will get not exactly the best outcomes from their work. Showing greatness currently will guarantee propensities for progress will convey forward.

8. STEPS BY STEPS INSTRUCTIONS TO KEEP A HABITS

Since it is now so obvious how to fabricate positive routines, we should investigate a few hints for you to keep up with your new way of behaving:

I. Establish a strong climate

Encircle yourself with similar individuals who have comparable objectives to you. Why? Since as people, we are significantly affected by what others around us are doing or feeling.

An investigation discovered that the effort of mental exertion is infectious. Basically doing an undertaking a great deal of close to an individual exertion will assist you with doing likewise.

Being around similar people is additionally uplifting. For instance, you might have framed a propensity for going for a disagreement the morning. Making associations with different sprinters will give you that additional energy and inspiration to adhere to your running propensities.

Being around a positive gathering who share comparable objectives and interests can be the single most noteworthy impetus to assist you with keeping up with your propensity.

Tell your family, companions, and partners what you will likely keep up with your new propensity. Sharing your propensity objectives gives responsibility and backing to your propensity upkeep.

2. Practice Self-empathy

It is challenging to Construct a propensity. In any case, keeping up with it might actually be seriously overwhelming.

Coming down on yourself to keep up with your propensity can be counterproductive. For instance, assuming that you neglect to stay aware of your propensity, zeroing in just on the failure can entice. Negative self-talk and programmed contemplations like "I've flopped once more" or "I won't ever succeed" will just hinder you.

All things considered, abstain from being excessively disparaging of yourself by rehearsing self-sympathy and close to home guideline. Advise yourself that propensity development and support is an excursion. What's more, disappointment is a characteristic piece of the excursion.

Try not to whip yourself, and spotlight on what future moves you can initiate.

3. Use Updates

One of the trickiest pieces of keeping a propensity is making sure to do it in any case. This is particularly evident when you're in the early phases of your propensity. As we've referenced above, it requires investment for activities to transform into ongoing ways of behaving.

To assist with keeping up with your propensity, set updates for yourself. This could be a visual update like a post-it on the cooler or your mirror.

Or on the other hand why not use innovation for your potential benefit? Set up updates on your telephone or download one of the many propensity following applications accessible. Some wearable pressure trackers and rest trackers have the usefulness to set updates.

You can likewise set updates about why you've chosen to focus on your new propensity, making you more propelled to keep focused and keep up with it.

9. CONCLUSION

Taking everything into account, growing positive routines doesn't need to be convoluted or scaring. With a tad of devotion and persistence, you can excel at building positive routines. Keep in mind, little changes and predictable exertion can go far. So be encouraged - take it each day and one propensity in turn. Best of luck!

www.ingramcontent.com/pod-product-compliance
Lightning Source LLC
LaVergne TN
LVHW052115160826
845678LV00015B/3572

9798374250442